Boobies 101

A Complete Guide to Breastfeeding for All Moms From a Mom

Written By

Heather Detmar

© Copyright 2014

Table of Contents

Introduction

Hi there,

I am a full-time working mother of five children, twin girls who are 16, two boys, 14 and 7, and a one-year old girl. I wrote this book to help other mothers get some insight and help on breastfeeding.

When I had my twins, I was 20 years old and had no clue what to do. I tried breastfeeding but was only successful with one of them, and that lasted for about a month before giving up. My older son was sick when he was born, so I was unable to breastfeed him, and my youngest son breastfed for about 3 months before I quit again. I was young and impatient, and had no guidance. With my last child, my youngest girl, I stuck to it. I bought a top of the line pump, spoke to a lactation consultant, and I have been going strong for a year now. My daughter and I have an incredible bond, far more than I had with my other children.

I must admit that at times it does get frustrating because she only wants me all the time, but heck, as I always say, "they are only little for a little while." Before I know it, she will be in high school like her sisters, so I take this time I have with her to relax, talk to her, and just enjoy my baby.

At first I was very embarrassed to feed or pump around anyone, even the nurses at the hospital, but slowly it stopped mattering so much and all I was concerned about was that my baby was hungry and I needed to feed her. Depending where I am I still may put a cover over myself, but I always feed her when she wants.

I went back to work when my baby was a little under three months old. Before that I pumped after every feeding for 15 minutes even if nothing came out as it helped stimulate my boobs. I continue to pump, even when I'm at work, two to three times a day to ensure she has enough milk when I'm not with her.

In the end, I know I am doing the best thing for my baby even when at times it can get overwhelming and frustrating. One regret I have is that I wish I was able to breastfeed all my children, but I am glad that it worked out with at least one of them. I wish you the best of luck on this new and wonderful journey you are about to embark on with your baby.

Good luck,

Heather

Chapter 1

Breastfeeding vs. Bottle-Feeding

It is no secret that breastfeeding is much more nutritious than traditional bottle-feeding. In this chapter I will discuss the pros and cons of breastfeeding versus those of traditional bottle-feeding.

Breastfeeding Pros

1. Breast milk contains a perfect balance of nutrients that your baby's body needs in order to grow and maintain perfect health.

2. Breast milk is something that is easily digested and absorbed by your baby's body.

3. Breast milk naturally changes to fit your baby's different changes in nutrition requirements.

3. It is 100% free, unlike formula, as your body naturally produces it and the only thing that you need to invest in is a breast pump and nursing pads.

4. Breast milk is always served at the ideal temperature and there is no risk of burning your baby.

5. You breast milk is available for your baby regardless of the time of the day.

Breastfeeding Cons

1. You are the only one who can feed your baby, unless you pump your milk and store it for times when you are not able to feed your baby by nursing.

2. You and your baby become dependent on each other. It may be hard for you to get away for any extended period of time. I was always hounded by the text messages "she won't stop crying," "come home," "the baby wants you."

3. It can be somewhat uncomfortable for new moms to breastfeed in public.

4. You have to watch what you eat and drink, as well as what medications you take. You may also find that your appetite increases greatly.

5. Breast milk digests faster than formula; therefore, you will most likely be the one getting up with your baby all through the night, as she or he will need to eat more often.

6. You may experience mastitis infections (infection of the breast tissue), clogged ducts, engorgement or discomfort, sore, cracked or bleeding nipples.

Bottle-Feeding Pros

1. Anyone you trust will be able to feed your baby.

2. You'll be able to tell exactly how much your baby is eating at each feeding.

3. It's more socially accepted to bottle feed in public.

4. New mothers can have more breaks and get more rest.

5. You won't have to be so concerned about the foods you eat or the medications you take.

Bottle-Feeding Cons

1. Newborn and Infant Formula only contain a few nutritious vitamins and minerals such as Vitamins A, C and D.

2. Many babies have difficulty tolerating certain formulas and some must even drink special formula so it doesn't irritate their stomachs.

3. You will spend approximately $100-$300 on formula alone to last the entire month as well as spend money on bottles and nipples.

4. You will have to take time to prepare each bottle before it can be given to your baby.

Chapter 2

Breastfeeding Basics

When it comes to breastfeeding some women find that there are days in which they are unable to produce the amount of milk that their baby needs and is craving for. There are a number of things that you can do to prepare your body for breastfeeding, and to create the milk you need so that the entire breastfeeding process is easier on you and your body.

Preparing Your Body for Breastfeeding

In order to prepare your body for breastfeeding, the first thing that you can do is try to educate yourself on breastfeeding alone as much as possible before your baby is even born. I even highly recommend taking a breastfeeding class where you can learn from other experienced mothers so that you will know what to expect when it comes time to breastfeeding your child. The more you prepare yourself to breastfeed, the more likely you will succeed at it and the less likely you will become easily frustrated.

However, there is really nothing else that you can do to prepare your body for breastfeeding. Whether you know it or not your body is already preparing itself for child rearing. The milk ducts and cells are working overtime to prepare your breasts to produce the milk you will need.

How to Breastfeed

While many people think that breastfeeding is one of the easiest things to do, that is not necessarily true. Sometimes a baby will nurse almost immediately while others will not. Some babies will be able to latch onto their mother's breast, others will not. Many times this can become quite frustrating to mothers as they do not know what else to do to get their baby to breastfeed. In this chapter we will go through step-by-step on how you breastfeed successfully and what you need to know about breastfeeding in general.

1. The very first thing that you do is to place your nipple between your baby's nose and upper lip. This helps to encourage your baby to open his or her mouth as you gently rub your nipple around his or her mouth. If this doesn't work for you try brushing the tip of your nipple against your baby's cheek. Your baby will naturally turn his or her head towards your breast and he or she will open her mouth to begin to suckle.

2. Once your baby begins to look for your breast with her mouth open (which is also known as rooting) encourage him or her to begin nursing by pulling him or her to your breast rather than bringing your breast to your baby.

3. The moment that your baby latches on, encourage him or her to get as much of your breast into his or her mouth. What this

does is encourage your baby to stay latched onto your breast and will give him or her the chance to nurse for as long as he or she can.

4. The best way to tell that you are breastfeeding correctly is when your baby's lips are opened wide around your breast and you feel no pain from it. You can tell that your baby is truly nursing when you hear him or her swallowing. If by chance you are feeling pain, break the connection slightly between you and your baby by sticking your finger on the side of the baby's mouth to help release and give it another try.

5. While your baby nurses try to hold him or her as close as possible. This allows your baby to feel your heartbeat and to remain calm as he or she feeds. This is also the time in which you can try to support your breast if it is large. You can also attempt to make yourself as comfortable as possible without jostling your baby and interrupting him or her during their feeding.

Remember, breastfeeding takes a lot of practice as well as patience before your baby is able to nurse without any problems. The key thing is to stay positive and remember, eventually the difficult part of breastfeeding will pass and you will be able to experience firsthand the natural joy that breastfeeding offers.

Breastfeeding Positions

While breastfeeding does require some practice and patience on your part, there are a variety of different positions that you can use in order to make the process easier on you. Here are a few positions that you can try and see if they will help make breastfeeding easier for both you and your baby.

1. **The Cross-Over Hold** - this position is also known as the cross-cradle hold. To use this position effectively choose which breast you want to nurse from, and support your baby with the opposite hand and arm. For example, if you are nursing from your left breast then take your right hand and arm to support your baby as he or she nurses. Next, rotate your baby's body until she is facing you and then use the fingers of your left hand to guide your baby to your breast. This hold is often used for babies who are smaller than usual and for those who have trouble latching onto your breast.

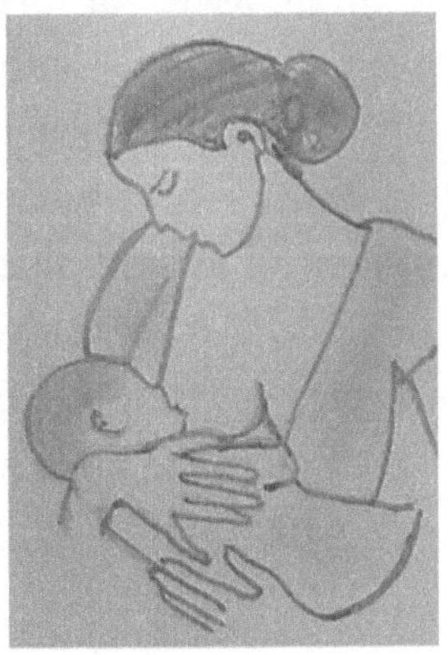

2. **The Traditional Cradle Hold** - this classic breastfeeding position, if used correctly, will have you cradle your baby's sensitive head in the crook of your arm. I highly recommend sitting in a chair with armrests or rest in a bed with comfortable pillows underneath your arm because after a few minutes your arm will start to become tired. In this position you will use the hand and arm that's on the same side as the breast you are nursing from. For example, if you are nursing from your left breast then you will use your left arm and hand to support your baby's body. Turn your baby's body until he or she is facing you and place his or her lower arm underneath their body and under your own arm. Make sure your baby's head rest in the crook at the elbow of your left arm. Next, use your right hand to guide your breast to your baby's mouth.

Your baby should be lying comfortably in a horizontal position. This position is most often used for babies who have been carried full-term. However, many mothers argue that this position makes it hard to help guide their baby's mouth to their nipple so do not feel embarrassed or ashamed if this hold does not work for you. Mothers who have had cesareans, such as myself, may find that this position causes pain on their abdomen. If you experience this, simply switch to a different position that is comfortable for you until your abdomen heals more.

-see image on next page

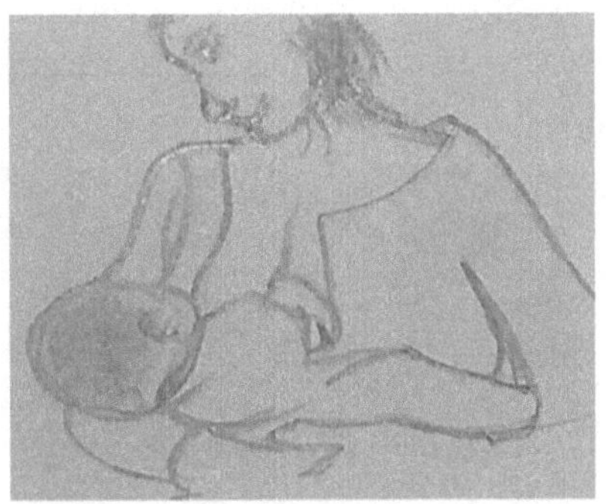

3. **The Football Hold** - just as the name implies, with this position you will need to hold your baby as you would hold a football. In this position you will need to tuck your baby under the arm that is on the same side as the breast you are going to be using. For example, if you're nursing from your right breast then use your right hand and arm to help support your baby's neck, head and shoulders, and slowly guide him or her to your nipple. Use your left hand to slightly lift your right breast out towards your baby's mouth.

When you use this hold you need to be extremely careful that you do not push your baby towards your breast so often that you will get him or her to resist it. Simply be gentle and remember to support his or her neck to prevent your baby from arching too much.

This position is commonly used by women who delivered their baby via cesarean, as their baby won't have to lie upon their stomach, and for women that have large breasts, flat nipples or those who deliver twins.

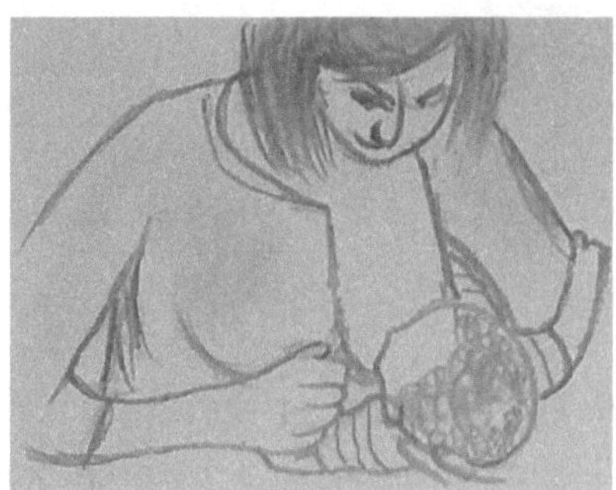

4. **The Reclining Hold** - when mothers use this hold they will need to be lying down and rolled onto their side so that their baby can easily reach their breasts. Surround yourself with a bunch of pillows, as it is important to keep your body in a straight line the entire time you breastfeed. Next, place your baby facing you and cradle your baby's head with your hand of the arm that is beneath you. For example, if you're lying on your left side then you will nurse from your left breast. Use your left arm to cradle your baby's head. If your baby is having trouble reaching you place a soft receiving blanket under his or her head in order to bring him or her closer to your breast.

16

This breastfeeding position can be used if you are recovering from having to deliver your baby via cesarean, or if you had an extremely difficult delivery that requires you to spend countless hours resting in bed.

Remember, each position can be used regardless of how you delivered your baby. If you find one hold that works for both you and your baby, stick with it. The key is to make sure that both you and your baby are comfortable when you breastfeed so that you can spend more time bonding with your child and less time being frustrated.

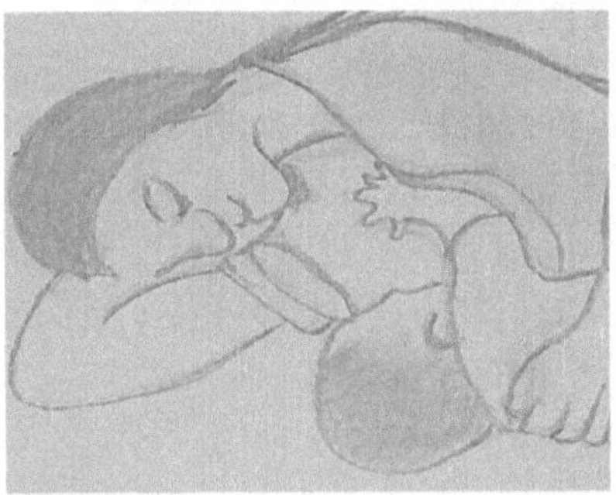

What Age Do You Stop Breastfeeding?

There are many healthy and nutritious benefits to breastfeeding your child. However, many mothers wonder when they should stop breastfeeding their child. The true answer to this is to stop breastfeeding when and only when you are ready, regardless of what your friends and family are telling you.

Remember, science is on your side. When you breastfeed your child for as long as possible you are providing your baby with many long-term health benefits such as preventing and lowering the risk of diabetes, heart disease and numerous nervous system disorders such as multiple sclerosis.

The decision is up to you. Trust your natural mothering instinct and make the decision that is best for both you and your baby.

Breastfeeding in Public

Many new moms may feel very uncomfortable with this practice, but don't let this be the deciding factor as to whether or not you'll breastfeed your baby. The benefits of breastfeeding your baby far out way this little fear, and rest assured that there are laws in place to protecting nursing moms.

There are many accessories to help conceal and make breastfeeding in public more comfortable for you, such as: nursing tops and dresses, breastfeeding blankets and breastfeeding slings.

Can I Get Pregnant While Breastfeeding

The answer is yes. You could start ovulating at anytime after three months of lactation, and your body will usually release its first postpartum egg before you being to menstruate again, so even though you are a lot less fertile you can still get pregnant. It is recommend to use some form of birth control, such as condoms, if you plan on having sex. Talk more with your doctor about other birth control options while breastfeeding.

What Foods Should I Avoid?

You don't have to be too picky with this one ladies, unless of course you have certain food allergies, or a family history of them. In general, you want to extremely limit your caffeine and alcohol intake, as well as fish that contain high levels of mercury and PCB's, such as Swordfish, Tilefish, Shark, Marlin and King Mackerel. Aside from this, feel free to indulge - variety is key!

I Am Sick, Should I Breastfeed?

Yes, you should absolutely continue to do so. Chances are that your baby was already exposed to these germs before you even became symptomatic. Although your baby will continue to be exposed while you breastfeed, this is also the best medicine for your baby because your breast milk is filled with the white blood cells and antibodies your baby needs to combat this illness.

One caveat, if you must take medication for your illness, then consult with you doctor because some medications can be harmful to your baby if your are breastfeeding.

Chapter 3

Breastfeeding Solutions

What to Do When Your Baby Won't Breastfeed

Some babies just don't get it. They try and try, but can't seem to latch on. This is not uncommon. My best piece of advice, don't quit! Some babies take longer than others to master the latch on. If this is happening with your baby, try some of these tips and techniques to help resolve the problem.

1. **Be persistent**-not forceful, but persistent. Keep trying with every feeding to get him or her to take your breast. Make sure to pump so that you have a supply of your milk to feed your baby until he or she learns to latch on properly. Plus the pumping will help your body to continue to produce milk even though your baby isn't quite nursing from your breast yet.

2. **Double check your positioning**. If this is the problem, you may have to take a trip to the doctor so that they can observe and help correct this.

3. **Try a nipple shield**. This is a soft little shield that is helpful when latch on problems occur. Typically made of silicone, this shield is used during breastfeeding and helps to hold the nipple in an extended position making it easier for the baby to suck the milk

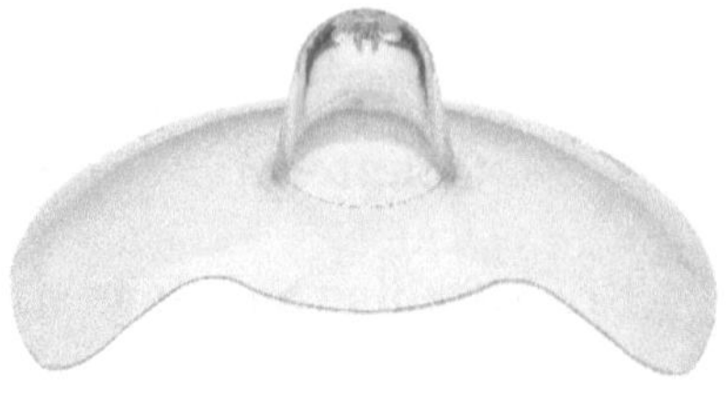

4. **Finger Feeding**. This method can help to train your baby to take your breast, and allows you to feed your baby without giving him or her an artificial nipple. You'll need a feeding bottle and a long thin tube (36 inches). Cut an enlarged hole into the tip of the nipple so that the tube can fit through it snugly. Fill the bottle with your breast milk or formula. Line the tube up with the inside of your middle or index finger. Use a small piece of medical tape and tape the tube to your finger. Gently place you finger inside your baby's mouth with the inside of your finger pointing towards the roof of your baby's mouth. Keep your finger as flat as possible to help keep your baby's tongue flat and forward. If you've done this correctly, your baby should start drinking.

-see image on next page

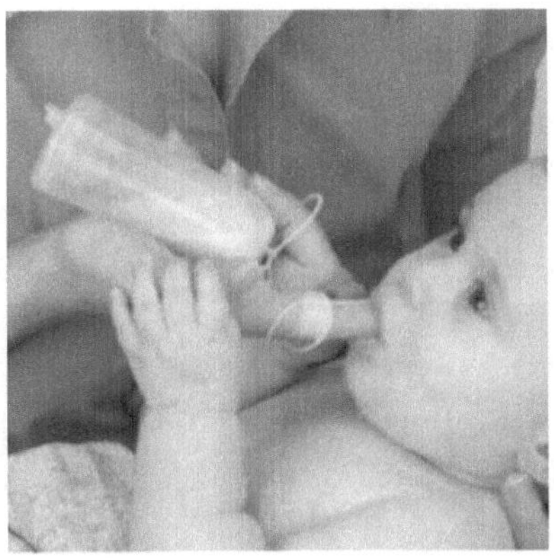

5. **Seek Professional Advice**. Take a trip to the doctor and discuss your concerns. Have your doctor fully exam your baby to make sure the issue is not a serious medical condition. Then discuss your options. Doctors are more familiar with these issues than you are and can usually come up with an effective solution. You may have to settle with bottle-feeding your baby with your breast milk or formula. You can also see a lactation consultant. They are in most hospitals and they can help you before you are discharged.

How To Create More Milk

When you are breastfeeding, sometimes you will feel as if you are not creating enough breast milk to satisfy your baby. You may even been wondering how you can help your body to create more milk so that you can satisfy your baby's needs. In this section you will learn a few ways that you can improve milk-let down (a term for the process where the nerves in your breasts send signals to release milk into your milk ducts) and have your body create more milk for your baby than you may need.

1. **Make sure that you take in enough calories during the day** - when you are breastfeeding it is crucially important that you take in no less that 1,800 calories a day and eat food that will be nutritious for both you and your baby. You would be surprised that what you take in can have a great impact on the amount of milk that your body produces. A few things that you should make sure you consume on a daily basis are calcium, plenty of fruits and plenty of vegetables, oatmeal, fenugreek vitamins, and almonds.

2. **Drink plenty of water** - if you are dehydrated; you will not be able to produce the milk that your baby needs. Because of this it is important to consume no less than six glasses of water daily.

3. **Pump your milk out several times a day** - you may be surprised to find that the more milk your body releases via a breast pump, the more milk your breasts will produce. The key to producing more milk for your baby is to pump at least 8 times during a 24 hour time period or to pump for about 15 minutes after your baby's feeding session.

Tip: Buy a high quality pump. It will make the process more efficient.

4. **Allow your baby to feed for as long as he or she wants -** while it is normal to feed your baby using a set schedule, in order to increase milk production allow your baby to feed for as long as he or she wants when you do feed him or her. This will help your breasts to produce more milk to fit your baby's needs.

Breastfeeding Supplies

In order to prepare yourself for the work that you will need to do when breastfeeding here is a list of supplies that I recommend you get for yourself. The more prepared you are, the easier breastfeeding will be for you and your baby.

1. **Nursing Bras** - while this is not required, I highly recommend that you invest in one of these. These kinds of bras are very comfortable to wear and will help to support your breasts especially when they are larger than usual. These bras are usually made with flaps that can easily come off when it is time to feed your baby.

Tip: If you do decide to go out and invest in a few of these bras, I recommend that you wait until the last couple of weeks during your pregnancy. The reason for this is because your breasts will be approximately the size they will continue to remain during the postpartum period.

2. **A Nursing Pillow** - this item will make feeding time more comfortable for your baby and for yourself. This kind of pillow

is one that wraps snugly around your waist area and is primarily used to help support your baby's weight while he or she is nursing. This pillow helps to keep you comfortable from straining your shoulders and neck during feedings and will help you to concentrate on bonding with your baby.

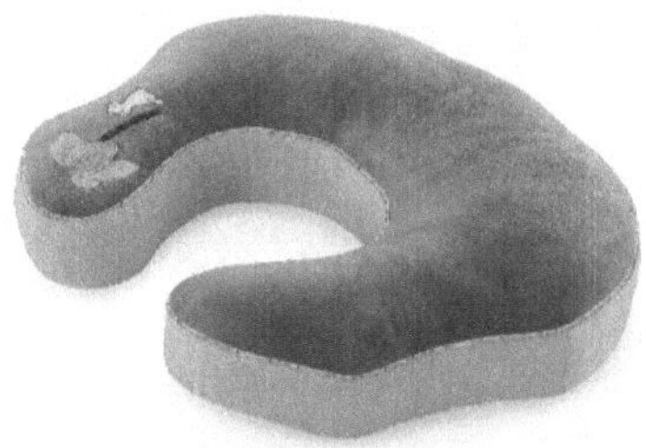

3. **Nursing Tops** - very similar to nursing bras, nursing camisoles and tops are made with convenient flaps that can be easily undone during feeding sessions and that can help give you and your baby some privacy. These work great when breastfeeding in public. Some of the nursing tops available today can also help to support your larger than normal breast size and can even act as a supportive bra if you need one.

-see image on next page

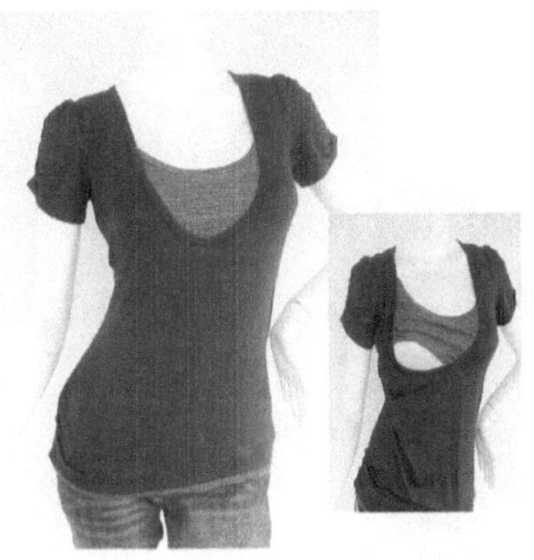

4. **Nursing Pads** - the reason why this item is on the list is because when you are breastfeeding it is normal for your breasts to leak some milk from time to time and anything such as seeing another baby can cause severe milk letdown. I recommend investing in a few disposable breast pads, as they will help keep your shirts looking dry and clean while you are out in public. You can find them is different shapes, colors, and patterns.

-see image on next page

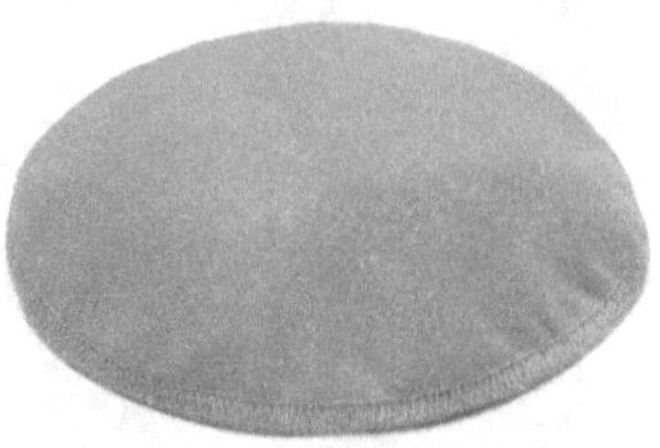

5. **A Breast Pump** - even if you do not think that you are going to pump your milk out regularly, a breast pump will come in handy especially if your breasts become painfully engorged. I will discuss more about breast pumps and how to choose one in Chapter 4.

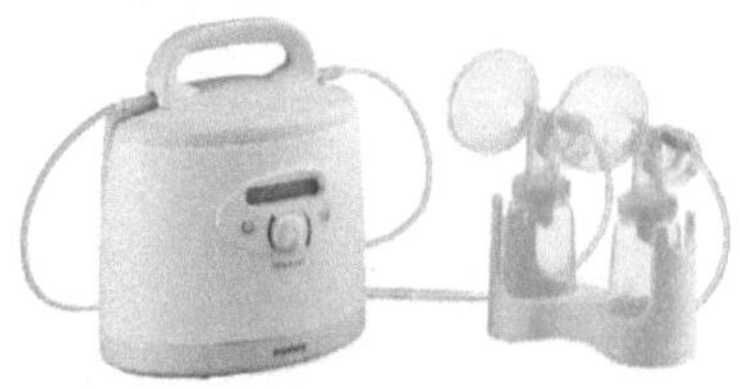

My Baby Hasn't Pooped, Is This Normal?

This can be completely normal. Your breast milk is so nutritious that your baby's body uses mostly all of it. Your baby can go a good week without having a bowl movement, but if it persists longer then this, or your baby is in pain, or straining, consult your   doctor.

Chapter 4

Breastfeeding Pumps

If you find that you are short on time and wish for your baby to still receive your breast milk, pumping is definitely the alternative you should consider. There are a variety of benefits to pumping your milk such as storing milk to use if you are not producing enough of it and reducing the chance of your breasts becoming painfully engorged. In this chapter you will learn how to use your breast pump to pump your milk, how to choose the right breast pump for you and how to store your breast milk.

Finding The Right Breast Pump For You

When it comes to finding the right breast pump to fit your needs, you may become overwhelmed by how many breast pumps there are available today. Here is a short list of a few things you should look out for when selecting a breast pump.

Note: I have found that the higher quality pumps can be very pricy; however, you may have the option to rent them as opposed to buying one out right. Check with your hospital or health insurance company to see if this option is available to you, and most health insurance will cover a pump.

1. **A Pump's Effectiveness** - one thing that you need to keep in mind is how effective a breast pump will be when pumping your milk. A baby has the ability to suck on your breast for about 45 to 55 times in a single minute. Look for a pump that can replicate this number, otherwise you may risk having sore nipples and ineffective pumping action.

2. **Types of Pumps Available** - there are a variety of different pumps that you can choose from. A single breast pump can be used for the occasional pumping as it can only be used on one breast at a time. This may be a good pump for stay at home moms or those that have a part-time job.

A double alternating pump is used to pump both breast using ample amounts of suction in order to force the milk out. This pump pumps both breasts at alternating times, but it is not as efficient as a double simultaneous pump.

A double simultaneous pump works the same as the other, but the difference is that it pumps both breasts at the same time. This pump is ideal for those who wish to cut their pumping time in half while increasing their overall milk production. I personally use a double simultaneous pump as I work a full-time job and I'm always tight on time.

3. **Motor Noise Level** - if you are the type of person who wants some discretion while they are pumping, you will need to find a

breast pump that makes little to no noise. Some moms really can't deal with the loud noise that hums from their pump. There are quality pumps on the market that are quieter, but they can be very pricy.

Tip: For a cheaper option, try placing your pump inside a tote bag and zipper is part way to help drown out the noise, or use a manual pump.

4. **Portability** - if you are working full-time, you will need to find a breast pump that will be easy to take with you. You can find a variety of pumps that are lightweight and that come with carrying bags that offer valuable discretion.

How To Use Your Breast Pump

Many mothers will claim that pumping your breast milk can be painful when that is not necessarily true. The reason as to why pumping breast milk is painful for many mothers is because they do not get a pump that is meant for their breast size or for their type of nipple. Once you start breastfeeding it is important to maintain a pumping and feeding schedule to reduce the chance of engorgement, which can be excruciating.

If you have never pumped your own breast milk, do not worry. You are not alone. In this section I have given you a step-by-step guide to make the process a little easier on you.

Step One: Find a quiet place where you can relax and be comfortable. Relaxing is a great way to help aid in milk let down and it also gives you a moment to yourself, without worrying about anything.

Step Two: You could use a warm compress or give your breasts a quick message to encourage your breasts to release milk. If your breasts are not responding to either of these, try having your baby nearby as this, more than anything, will help cause your milk to be released.

Step Three: Bring the pump up to your breasts and insert your nipple into the suction cup. Ensure that your nipple fits snuggle within the opening and rests comfortably around your breasts.

Step Four: Turn on the pump on low suction first. The reason why you want to start with the lowest suction possible is to give your breasts adequate time to begin releasing enough milk. Once your milk begins to flow, increase the suction.

Step Five: Sit back and relax as the pump goes to work. You want to pump for at least 15 minutes to be able to store enough milk for your baby later on.

The Best Time to Pump Breast Milk

While breastfeeding you may find yourself pumping throughout the day in order to keep up with your baby's demand for milk.

However, is there really a time of the day that is better for you to pump than any other time? In fact, there is.

The best time for any mother to pump her breasts is right before her baby wakes up in the morning. Always begin at least an hour to two hours before your little one wakes or you can pump while she is feeding from one of them. The reason why it is more effective to pump your breasts in the morning is simply because while you have rested throughout the night, your breasts have been stockpiling the milk inside of you the entire time. Once you pump first thing in the morning, you will find that you will be able to pump more ounces than you are accustomed to and thus will be able to store more milk for your baby in the months to come.

It's important to note that you must pump regularly, in addition to breastfeeding, throughout the day every day. The reason for this is because if you are not breastfeeding or pumping enough, you run the risk of your breasts becoming blocked. This is known as a Blocked Milk Duct, and occurs when one of your ducts becomes partially obstructed. If this happens, it will form a lump, and if not treated quickly and properly, it can turn into an infection. If you're a mom who produces a lot of milk, you are especially prone to this.

Tip: To help combat a milk duct that is blocked, try feeding your baby on the affected side for consecutive feedings. I found that warm compresses, hot showers and soft massages to the blocked area also help.

Storing Your Breast Milk

Today there are many different breast pumps available that come with custom made containers where you not only collect the breast milk that has been pumped, but that you can use to store your breast milk. You can also use specially made breast milk storage bags, which you can find almost anywhere. You can place your breast milk in your refrigerator only if you plan to use it within an eight to twenty-four hour period; otherwise place it in your freezer where you can store it for up to six months, or one year in a deep freezer.

If you plan on freezing your breast milk I recommend that you only store up to three or four ounces in one container at a time. You will want to do this because it will allow for an easier time thawing and to allow for expansion. To keep track of all of the containers you will undoubtedly have in your freezer, label each container you have with the date and time it was pumped and be sure to use the oldest containers of breast milk first.

Chapter 5

Breastfeeding Twins or More

About 1 in every 30 births in the United States is twins, and 1 in every 726 births is triplets or more. You may feel that you have no idea how you will handle breastfeeding twins, or if you'll produce enough milk, have enough time, or enough energy to keep up. All of these are valid concerns, but trust me, with proper planning and help from loved ones breastfeeding twins can be successfully done. I know, because my very first pregnancy was twin girls; therefore, let me try to clear up some of your concerns.

Will I Have Enough Time?

Time wise, it will take roughly about the same amount of time to breastfeed twins as it would to bottle-feed, actually maybe longer to bottle-feed since you have to sterilize the bottles and warm the formula. It's best to keep a flexible feeding schedule because both babies may not want to feed at the same time. This is okay, don't force them, just let them dictate their feeding schedule.

Tip: If your babies end up eating on different schedules, try pumping the unused breast during the feeding to help keep up your milk production.

If both your babies want to feed at the same time, no worries, just use your nursing pillow for support (they make ones especially for twins) as this will help free your hands to help position and further support your babies. The traditional cradle (A) and football-clutch (B) holds work best with twins in this position.

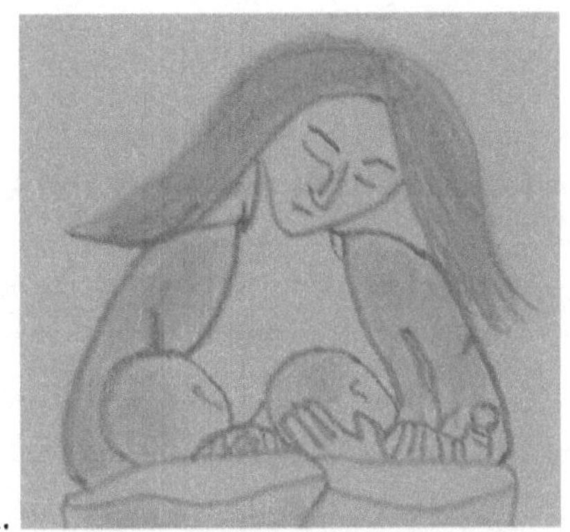

A.

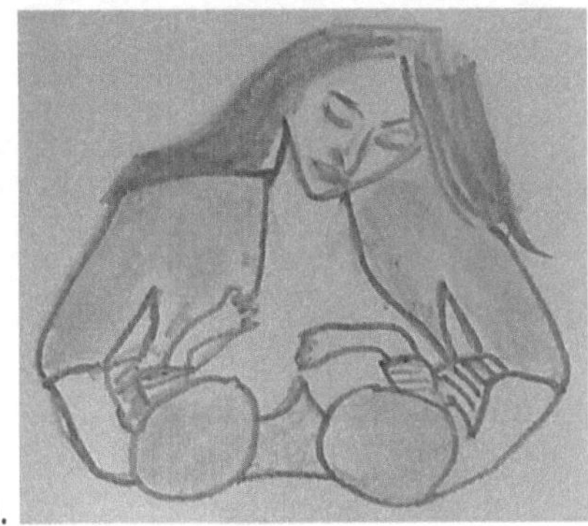

B.

Tip: Try alternating your breast each baby feeds on about every 24 hours. This will help to produce equal amounts of milk in each breast and give the babies added stimulation.

If you feel that you need a break and some much need rest, ask your partner or family members for help. One of the great things about pumping is that you can store extra breast milk that can later be put into a bottle, allowing others to feed the babies while you take a break.

How Will I Breastfeed My Twins When I'm Out and About?

Don't stress yourself out with this one. Yes, it is harder to breastfeed your twins at the same time when you're out in public, especially without your nursing pillow and props. My best suggestion to you, and what worked best for me, is to breastfeed them one at a time. If they are already on separate schedules, this will work nicely for you. If they're used to eating at the same time, feed one right after the other.

Your partner or support team can come in very handy here because they can help keep one baby occupied while you feed the other.

Will I Produce Enough Milk for Two?

Trust in Mother Nature. Our bodies are equipped to supply us with whatever we need. If you do find that your running low on milk, try feeding or pumping more often. This will help you to produce more.

Make sure you take your babies to the doctor for regular checkups to ensure that both of them are eating properly and getting an adequate supply of milk.

Added Support

If your support system is scarce and you need additional resources and or information then the La Leche League International (LLLI) is a great place to turn. The LLLI is an international organization that provides support and information to breastfeeding mothers. You can go to their website and search for a support group in your area.

Breastfeeding Triplets or More

I personally have not had the experience of having triplets; however, I can tell you that a lot of the information in my book can be applied to nursing triplets or more.

In addition, there is an organization called The Triplet Connection that is a great resource for moms expecting triplets or more, plus keep in mind that the LLLI can help you find additional resources as well, and can put you in touch with mothers who have gone through this experience.

Chapter 6

Breastfeeding When You're Diabetic

If you're an expecting mother living with type 1 or 2 diabetes, you may be wondering if you can breastfeed and how it will affect your baby. I do not have diabetes, but I have done a fair amount of research on the subject, and can offer you some rich insight.

Can I Breastfeed If I Have Diabetes?

Yes, you most definitely can, and you should. You must however, closely monitor your diet to keep your condition regulated, albeit it has been documented that some mothers actually require less insulin during lactation.

Additional Facts About Breastfeeding When Your Diabetic

1. Your milk may take a few days longer to come in then that of a healthy mother without diabetes.

2. Breastfeeding your baby will lower their risk of developing diabetes.

3. It can help moms lose weight.

4. It can help your body use insulin more effectively.

5. It can lower your body's need for insulin.

6. It can help mothers feel emotionally and physically better.

Gestational Diabetes

This is a form of diabetes that affects women during their pregnancy even though they may have never had diabetes before. It's estimated that about 4 percent of expecting mothers will develop this condition. Experts say that the condition will disappear after childbirth; however, you are more likely to develop it again with future pregnancies, and there are cases where mothers who developed gestational diabetes actually develop type 2 diabetes later on in life.

The Process of Gestational Diabetes

Let me further explain exactly what is happening with gestational diabetes. Basically, people with diabetes have excessively high amounts of sugar in their blood. Normally, your digestive system breaks down your food into glucose (a type of sugar), then the glucose goes into your blood stream and is converted into fuel with the help of insulin, which is a hormone produced by your pancreas. In people with diabetes, their pancreas isn't producing enough insulin to convert all the glucose to fuel; therefore, too much glucose remains in their blood.

Gestational Diabetes will develop in pregnant women who's hormonal changes are requiring their body's to create more insulin then their pancreas can produce; therefore, the blood glucose level rises and results in gestational diabetes. Since this condition is caused by hormonal changes due to pregnancy, once a woman gives birth and her hormone levels revert back to normal the gestational diabetes will disappear.

Additional Facts About Gestational Diabetes

1. Gestational diabetes usually has no symptoms; therefore, it's recommended that expecting mothers have a glucose screening test.

2. You're at higher risk if: you're obese, had gestational diabetes in the past, have a family history of it, you have high blood pressure, you're over 35, gave birth to a baby with defects, have sugar in your urine.

3. There is treatment for it so you can deliver a healthy baby.

4. Your doctor may want to induce labor early or suggest a cesarean to prevent any delivery problems.

Chapter 7

Medications, Drugs and Alcohol:
What You Need To Know

Medications

When you breastfeed, the most important thing that you have to remember is that whatever you eat, drink or take into your body will be passed on to your baby when they feed. That is why it is especially important to watch everything that you take into your body, especially medication. There are a variety of medications that can be passed onto your baby and that can even affect your overall milk supply and you need to be wary of them. If you are in doubt be sure to talk with your baby's doctor and research thoroughly before taking any medication that could prove harmful.

Drugs and Alcohol

The same goes for any drugs or alcohol that you may take. If you use drugs recreationally you cannot do so if you plan on breastfeeding. Remember trivial drugs such as marijuana and cocaine can pass through your milk and affect your baby in such a way that it can prove to be potentially fatal; therefore, it is highly advised that you refrain from using any illicit drugs while breastfeeding.

The risks are not as clearly defined when it comes to consuming alcohol while breastfeeding as opposed to during pregnancy. The more alcohol you consume the longer it takes for it to be eliminated from your body, and the effects it will have on your baby are directly related to the amount of alcohol you drink. Alcohol will completely pass through the mother's system. Again, how long that takes depends on the amount of alcohol consumed. Generally speaking, it takes about one hour to eliminate a .016 level of alcohol (.016 BAC is equal to one serving of beer or wine). This timeframe can vary depending on a person's height, weight, and body fat percentage.

If you must drink, then it is best to wait until the alcohol is out of your system before you start breastfeeding again. You can try to pump out 24 hours worth of clean breast milk that your baby is going to need. Then drink. However, your baby should not drink from you until the alcohol leaves your system, and during this time I recommend that you pump your breasts anyway, but do not store the milk you produce. Instead, toss it out as it may be contaminated with the alcohol you consumed. Once the alcohol is out of your system, then you can freely breastfeed as you had before. You can purchase from a convenience store what's known as milkscreen test strips to measure the amount of alcohol in your breast milk.

Cigarettes

Should you breastfeed if you're a cigarette smoker? Yes, you can and you most likely should. Ideally, you should give up the habit, and not just for your baby, but for yourself. However, as I mentioned before, breast milk is so nutritious that if you're a smoker breastfeeding is one of the ways to help your baby fight off some of the effects that cigarette smoking can have on them, especially their lungs.

Some things you should be aware of if you're a smoker and can't give up the habit. The nicotine that transfers into your breast milk can upset your baby. It can also lower your ability to produce milk and interfere with milk let-down. Babies who are exposed to second-hand smoke are more likely to suffer from pneumonia, asthma, bronchitis, eye irritation, ear infections, sinus infections, croup and colic. It increases their chances of respiratory infections, allergy-related illnesses and sudden infant death syndrome (SIDS), and can significantly lower their HDL cholesterol levels.

So moms, if you can't quit altogether, then consider cutting down on the amount of cigarettes you smoke per day, and avoid smoking in the same room as your baby. This goes for dads too! Don't smoke right before or during breastfeeding, and wait as long as possible between smoking and nursing.

Is It Safe To Get A Tattoo While You Are Breastfeeding?

You would be surprised how often this question is asked. Why wouldn't it be? If nearly everything that you take into your body can be transferred to your baby via your milk, why wouldn't tattoo ink?

In fact, tattoo ink is one of the few things that will not be transferred to your baby via your breast milk. Tattoo ink is safe because it is only used on your skin. It will not go into your blood circulation where it has the chance to get into your breast milk.

However, the one thing that you will need to be fearful of is the needle used by the tattoo artist itself. You need to ensure that you visit a tattoo shop that uses ethical practices and clean tattooing because if you're tattooed by a used needle, you risk contracting Hepatitis B, Hepatitis C, HIV and other blood-born diseases.

Tip: Be wary and stay away from tattoo artist who only tattoo out of their house. Unless they are a well-known artist running a legit shop from their home, I highly suggest going a tattoo shop as they are regulated by the state and are enforced to use clean practices, and their artist are required to be licensed by the state (these laws may vary state to state, so be sure to check up on your state's laws regarding the operations of tattoo shops).

You can rest assured that the chance of that happening is slim to none. It has been proven that you are more likely to contract

46

these harmful diseases at a dentist office than you are at a tattoo shop. However, it is still something that should always remain in the back of your mind.

Conclusion

Thank you again for buying this book! I hope it has given you some insight on breastfeeding, and if you learned one thing I am happy because I really did not know much about breastfeeding until my fifth child. It all seems very overwhelming, but in the end all you really need to do is be there for your baby, your body will do the rest.

I have provided an email address below should you have any questions. I am not a doctor, but I will do my best to answer them. Also, if you enjoyed this book, please take the time to share your thoughts and post a review on the site you bought the book from. If it didn't meet your expectations, then let me know your suggests for improvement. My goal is to make this the most complete affordable guide to breastfeeding that any mom will ever need.

Best of luck to you, and congratulations on your new baby!

Thank you,

Heather Detmar

heatherdetmar@yahoo.com